I0709794

THE AFFECTION PRESCRIPTION: 7 steps to more intimate connection, love and joy

TABLE OF CONTENT

CHAPTER ONE

KEEP IN TOUCH

Even if you live together, stay together, or share a bed, it is essential to be in touch regularly in a romantic relationship. Maintaining in touch or making contact goes deeper than merely seeing each other's faces every day in the home.

But before you can know and comprehend love and devotion, you must first get to know the one who represents love. According to the Bible, "God is love, and whoever does not love does not know God."

You must understand that the love and affection we're discussing came from God and that He is love; otherwise, you won't be able to love as He intended until you do.When you comprehend the circumstances under which God chose to offer humanity love, you realize that it wasn't because we were pure or pleasant to Him on earth before

He gave us love; rather, He made the decision to bestow His care on people despite their severe wickedness and rebellion. In order to save us from sin and everlasting punishment, he sent his only son, Jesus Christ, to earth to come and die on the cross. All of us who are saved and washed by the blood of Jesus today would have been lost along with the rest of the world if God had waited for mankind to please or love Him before He carried out the plan to redeem us. However, God's compassion for mankind was great and is still great today, even when we are lost in sin. "Christ died for us while we were still sinners." He first loved us, so now that he has, we also love him. We are in contact with Him and He with us because He removed the barrier that was standing between us—sin—and gave us the opportunity to be personal with Him once again.Since sin's hold over us has been destroyed, we are now able to serve God without being afraid of death or the ravages of this world.

For you to realize and appreciate the truth that
everyone today who has a connection with God
is based on love and that relationship is
maintained by love, I've chosen to start this way.
It is a romantic connection. If we don't approach
our connection with God with this knowledge, it
won't be healthy for us to become closer to him.
I realize that everyone must be led to God by His
spirit, but you are still expected to answer when
He calls out to you since it is a love language,
and because it is love and not force, He will
leave you alone if you don't. You must fully
comprehend this, otherwise it will be difficult
for you to stay in touch with God, who is love,
and your responses to Him will be based on your
feelings of love for Him. Even if what He asks
you to do seems tough and silly to others, and
even if everyone else is backing away, you
won't, because you are connected to Him by a
chord of love, and you won't. (Rom 5:5 Hope
does not produce shame because the holy spirit
that is given to us causes the love of God to be
diffused widely in our hearts. You can only love
like God when the Holy Ghost bestows this sort

of love on your heart. Therefore, God sends you the Holy Spirit when you become a new creation, and one of the things the Holy Spirit accomplishes in our hearts is bring the love of God, the same love that the Father had in His heart that moved him to release His only begotten Son to come and die to save the world. Because of his intense love for the flawed, sinful world, he was unable to withhold him. Instead, he had to show him. (John 3:16)

This implies that serving Him and following Him will no longer be a struggle, and obeying Him won't be difficult or painful. Keep my commandments if you love me. Our obedience to His commands demonstrates our love for Him, just as His sending His Son to save the world demonstrated His love for us.

Our amount of affection for him is strongly correlated with our obedience. Whether or not he is the first in your life depends on how yielding you are. Your adherence to his rules and instructions not only indicates to the world around us how much you love him.

This is crucial to understand before I discuss the topic of communication because it is normal for anyone who has not gone through the death of the old man, the expulsion of the old nature of sin, and the termination of the flesh and self-life to be selfish in their relationships with others, including their spouse. It is not your fault that you were born that way; rather, it is a result of the wicked adamic nature that has existed since the fall of man in Ede. This is the nature that all of us were born with by our original parents. There is only one way to cope with this evil nature—a selfish, rebellious, and sinful nature—and that is through the death of Jesus Christ on the cross. This wicked nature could not be destroyed in any other way.

This nature exists in every person who has not accepted the cross of Christ, where the old nature was dealt with; you need to allow God to assist you right now while you are reading this information. If you continue in this manner, you will not be able to experience love. Instead, allow Jesus to enter your life right away and you will discover a new kind of love. Please don't let today's chance pass you by once again. He has been seeking you and is waiting with open arms and compassion to welcome you. Can you stop right now and start praying, telling him that you are prepared to submit to him and that you really mean it? Ask him to purify you with his blood, complete in your life what he started on the cross, and record your name in the Lamb's Book of Life.

If you feel that the aforementioned has been completed, you may continue or go on; if not, kindly stop. I'm grateful. The first and most crucial person to maintain an uninterrupted connection with is God, leading to that closeness with the holy spirit. The advantages, fragrance, and scent of your connection with God will be used in other human relationships, including your marriage. This implies that your devotion to your connection with God will serve as the foundation for all other relationships and your treatment of others. Since God will correct you and require that you make amends, you won't anger or offend them. But if you don't, you'll be doing it at the risk of your connection with Him. It is crucial to start your love life with God and be anchored in Him since this is why it is a love relationship. Nobody wants to insult or dishonor the person they love. He is the first person you can always stay in contact with and maintain a close friendship with.

CHAPTER TWO
DISCOVER THE SECRET

Discovering something involves exposing it or removing its cover. It also means revealing something that has been concealed or unknown in the past. In order to properly appreciate what was hidden, it must be brought to light.

This can be accomplished using a variety of techniques, including conducting a study and distributing questionnaires; if the purpose of your study is more external, such as for a college project, a business project, a survey, environmental surveillance, and more; you can also gather information from various sources to form your results; other people use the inspection method, in which people are deployed into the environment to interact with local residents on a regular basis. Deeply researched decisions often have compelling evidence behind them.

Contrarily, a secret is anything that is kept secret or even private. Secrets may be beneficial or detrimental, good or evil.

As was previously said, there are several ways that individuals find secrets. These methods vary from person to person and from organization to organization, and they are often appropriate for the institution involved. Since education aims to develop children's minds and intellects while the police are tasked with maintaining public safety, for instance, educational institutions won't adopt police practices. Additionally, the techniques used by the spouses in a marriage vary.

Get to Know Your Spouse

We shall now focus on a smaller number of methods of discovery in order to better serve the goals of this book.

Research has repeatedly demonstrated that even though many people are married, living together, and sharing a bed, they still don't know one another well enough to be married for years while being complete strangers. The fact is that the premarital counseling and other premarital programs you took, together with the premarital search you conducted, are all excellent and highly recommended for anybody who intends to fulfill the God-designed goal of marriage. However, if you have made any findings before, your study will continue while you are married in order to learn more about your spouse.

I want to emphasize once again how crucial it is to pay attention to the truth from the previous chapter because it is essentially going to help you navigate throughout this trip. In the same way that he led you into it, God will continue to guide you through your marriage in the same way. Your connection with God comes first, and that includes all other relationships you may have, including your marriage. Your relationship with the God who created you will be where you learn the most about yourself.

Concerns about knowing your partner that are externally connected This will allow me to identify certain opportunities and explain how to successfully utilize them. The goal is to gradually increase your level of closeness with your partner.

Pose inquiries.

Asking your partner questions in a loving manner is one of the most effective ways to get to know them better. Without making thoughtful, respectful inquiries, you will simply be dealing with assumptions if you undertake any kind of research. Even if it's a positive or negative action or response, don't presume it to be something else; instead, please ask questions and learn to speak about it. You don't know him or her by assumption. Assuming you are familiar with your spouse, it may be highly expensive. With the creation of this platform, you will learn more about your spouse.

regular interaction.

Communication in any kind of relationship, including marriage, is one of the key components to enhancing and making intimacy attainable and simple. When there are sufficient avenues of communication, customers may provide accurate feedback and replies that can assist in meeting their demands. Understanding communication and heart-to-heart communion are what keep marriages strong. Most of your questions will arise at this point because you and your spouse have such a strong emotional connection that you can really look into one another's hearts. Don't overlook this part of the prescription; it's crucial to building closeness. When there is a lack of communication with your spouse, he or she may opt to confide in someone else rather than you or, worse yet, to remain silent and endure the suffering alone, which may be harmful. So, regardless of how effective it is, don't allow your line of communication to get cut off for any reason.

You are not merely interested in learning about your spouse's eccentricities and, certainly, being against them, as some individuals will or are currently doing. But it's the realization of his or her whole self. This will support you in your quest for closeness and kinship. You two are designed to complement one another in every way while you work on each other. Maintain your passion, love, and devotion for one another.

You must be diligent in this process; it requires meticulous research to bring out the person's hidden assets for the sake of your relationship.

And if you learn anything strange about your spouse throughout the process, it would be best not to use it against them. God sees everyone as a work in progress. You may brag to the world about your spouse's qualities, but please keep his or her flaws to yourself and seek to correct them as you respectfully discuss how to manage them.

CHAPTER THREE
APPRECIATION

The act of appreciating something is based on your understanding of its value, weight, and significance. It is a reward for excellence. It means expressing gratitude or gratitude for anything. Therefore, it is necessary to appreciate one another in a marriage with extraordinary understanding.

Your understanding of them will serve as the basis for an adequate act of gratitude;

How important are they to you?
The value of that person in your life is
How special a person is to you.

A profound grasp of a thing's worth, value, and significance to you, your family, and the environment is necessary for appreciation to develop.

For instance, when there is nothing to eat at home or when you are even utterly destitute, realizing that God gave you the breath in your nostrils and that you are the reason he never sleeps or slumbers should make you feel grateful and appreciative of him.

Being God is not only a result of his goodness; it is who he is. Day and night, he is devoted to protecting us.

One day I was thinking about the verse in Palms 121:4 that says, "Behold, he who maintains Israel never slumbers or sleeps." And it dawned on me that I am the reason the Almighty God would not sleep or rest because He made it his personal responsibility to watch over me so zealously for as long as I live and dwell in Him, rather than just for a day, month, or year.the same forever and every day. I recently burst into unceasing gratitude and admiration for who he is, his magnificent accomplishments, and many other things just thinking about this alone. Only individuals with profound thinking abilities are able to continuously express gratitude. Deep reflection on God's kindness leads to appreciation.

This is why you need to get to know your spouse because you won't know how to appreciate her more if you don't have a stróng feeling of her worth and value. When you realize what a blessing and how much of a help he or she is to you, you will be thankful to God for him or her. Money or material possessions are not the only things a woman needs to be a successful wife and mother at home; it goes beyond just purchasing her stuff. Your expression of gratitude must touch all aspects of your spouse's life.

The majority of the time, it's not the large things you do, but rather how exceptional you make the small things appear that might address an emotional need.

When you learn to appreciate your spouse more, he or she will feel more free to be who they are supposed to be. Your understanding of your partner as who you have come to know them to be will give rise to an unending amount of appreciation. You will be grateful for all he does before you even see what he or she accomplishes.

Enjoy every moment you have together.

CHAPTER FOUR
MUTUAL RESPECT AND HONOR

Since this is born out of a profound feeling of worth and value put on your partnership with him or her, there have been many things said in the early chapters of this book about honour and respect in marriage.

Therefore, demonstrating respect implies you value all your partner contributes to the table, including their qualities, abilities, eccentricities, and prior experience. Your individuality has worth. Mutual respect allows people to be who they really are without worrying about being judged. Because you are both unique creations, embrace your differences and avoid comparing yourselves.

Give room

Recognizing certain needs shows you have respect for one another. As a result, you may need to establish limits and decide what you need to recharge and renew. This can include allowing one another some distance. Space might be defined as giving your spouse a kiss when they get home, not pressuring them to speak about their day, or not putting pressure on them when they want to go out with friends. Allowing solitude or time with others while not hovering demonstrates maturity and respect. It is crucial that you and your spouse maintain supportive connections outside of marriage to meet your social demands.

Encourage each other.

Encourage your partner to know that you love and respect them. Putting your effort and attention towards speaking life over your spouse will show them that you value and respect them as a person. Being your spouse's biggest supporter is a good idea. By recognizing one another's accomplishments and encouraging one another when the going gets rough, we can champion one another. Never criticize your partner in front of relatives or friends. If you have issues with your partner, it is impolite to speak poorly about them. The same is true if you disagree with your spouse in front of other people. By supporting your spouse, you are maintaining your unity and being on the same team.

A marriage may eventually get stronger as a result of respect; the more consistent you are, the stronger it will be. sincerely love and take pleasure in honoring one another.

According to what the Bible says, Christians should respect or honor all men (1 Peter 2:17). We must appreciate and cherish the fact that every human being carries the imprint of God. All in all, the Bible also commands us to love our neighbor (Leviticus 19:18), and Jesus emphasizes the point in his well-known parable that our neighbor is anyone God has put in front of us (Luke 10:29–37). Therefore, all Christians are expected to love and respect all people. That forms the foundation.

But Scripture places a significant, extra focus on the unique connection between husbands and wives and between women and husbands. In particular, husbands are commanded to love their spouses as Christ loved the church (Ephesians 5:25). The church particularly instructs wives to appreciate their husbands as Christ respects the church (Ephesians 5:33).

We should remember three things as a result of this. Although there are more teachings than just these three, we should strive to understand at least these three.

Love and respect are our duties.

Women who are cherished by their husbands will become more beautiful. A husband who is appreciated by his wife will get greater respect. First, the directives are focused on our individual and comparative areas of weakness. We are instructed to carry out actions that we may not carry out on our own. For instance, children are instructed to follow their parents since it is simple for them to do otherwise (Ephesians 6:1). Similar to this, it is advised for men to adore their spouses since it is simple for them not to. Because it is simple for women to neglect their husbands, ladies are advised to do so. The things we are asked to perform may not occur to us. Why bring it up if we were all doing these things naturally?

Men are not as good at love as women are. Men are good at showing respect. According to C.S. Lewis, women see love as going through hardship for others, which is considerably more in line with the biblical model of agape love than what males often do. Men often equate love with not causing difficulties for others.

Men must thus be urged to make sacrifices and go through hardships for their spouses, just as Christ did for the church. It is necessary to nudge women to respect their spouses. Paul would consider it problematic for a woman to love a man who is not highly respected or honored in her eyes. How many times have we heard a heartbreaking tale of a girl who, despite her abusive boyfriend's treatment of her, keeps going back to him because she "loves" him? The response she would give if we asked her whether she respected him is, "Are you kidding? Him? " Additionally, males must be called upon to abandon themselves for their spouses. What a Marriage entails is this.

Women run on love, men on respect.

Second, the command provides information about the recipient's requirements. In other words, it would be logical to assume that sheep need food if the Bible instructed shepherds to feed their flock. We may conclude that women must be cherished if husbands are instructed to do so. We may conclude that husbands must be respected if women are to be taught to do so. Imagine two distinct automobile types, such as

diesel and normal, using various types of fuel.
Wives run on love, while men run on respect.

"Stuff your partner's appreciate. On respect, men
thrive. Love sustains women.
Keep in mind that we are discussing emphasis
when you hear me say this. Everyone needs to
be loved and appreciated on the most
fundamental level. But when Scripture
specifically mentions married couples living
together, it commands men to love and women
to respect. Turn this back, and you'll realize that
husbands must respect their wives just as much
as ladies must remember that their husbands
must cherish them.

By keeping this in mind, we are able to avoid
giving instead of receiving. According to a
saying by George Bernard Shaw, we should not
treat people as we would want them to treat us,
since their preferences may not be the same as
ours. A guy I once knew gave his wife a lovely
shotgun for Christmas. The next Christmas, she
gave him a lovely strand of pearls since she was

a cunning Christian lady. And she said, "They were extremely lovely pearls," as she said to my wife.

When a marriage is having trouble, both partners often offer what they believe they need from the other—love and respect, respectively. When respect would be more beneficial, wives tend to reach out to their husbands with affection. When what is needed is a deep embrace of affection, husbands may choose to pull away while believing that this is a sign of respect or "providing space."

Both have the ability to bring about change.

Thirdly, though, and here is where things really shine, love and respect are both strong. This sort of love is effective, according to what the Bible says. This level of respect is strong. This kind of love bestows beauty. Respect in this nature bestows respectability.

Women see love as causing problems for others, but men often view love as not causing trouble for others.

The kind of love that made Christ's bride beautiful and which husbands cannot equal
While we were still sinners (Romans 5:8), Christ died for us. Husbands are advised to emulate this type of love even if they are unable to replicate it. We also see some of the same results when we copy it. A wife who is cherished by her husband will become more beautiful with time. He cleans her with the Word's water (Ephesians 5:26). The whole paragraph is predicated on the idea that this type of love bestows beauty. The regard of a virtuous woman also has the same type of power. Peter explains that a man's wayward spirit may be crushed by respectful and chaste conduct (1 Peter 3:1–2).

Men and women should therefore respect and love one another. They need to put all their heart into it. But the guys should lean into love while they are focusing on their relationships. The

ladies need to lean toward respect. The outcomes
might be astounding.

CHAPTER FIVE

ACKNOWLEDGE AND SAY I'M SORRY

I'm sorry is not a language of the weak but of the strong; it is not just spoken when one is wrong but also when one values the person to whom the apology is being made.
The one who offers an apology first is just expressing how much they valued the friendship.

Many people are too big to say "I'm sorry," but the reality is that you are huge and proud, which is the attitude of an egotistical person.

As you gain closeness, you must learn to express your regret verbally rather than through the deplomatic technique of compensating by purchasing something special. Even if you purchase things, you still need to apologize when you are wrong since connection and bonding need it. You will learn that there is just you and your partner against everything as your connection with one another grows.

Be aware that your spouse may not take offense from other sources seriously since this is the way the world is. The world may turn against you and your marriage, but as long as your love and understanding are still there, you will be able to overcome this. However, when an offense occurs inside the marriage, it generally hurts more deeply since it comes from the person you love. I did not anticipate such from him or her, and he or she ought to have understood what I like and don't like, which are common phrases.

But after all of that, practice saying "I'm sorry" to people since it cures wounds more quickly than any medication in existence.

I'm sorry conveys a sense of duty, affection, and concern. It demonstrates that you love, care for, and are in charge of everything required to keep the two of you together. Please take it in.

How to Use "I'm Sorry" to Strengthen Your Marriage

You can sincerely tell that something is wrong with you. That insulting comment still hurts. A promise that will not be fulfilled today passes the time. There are different loyalties, and your spouse places you at the bottom of their list. Due to the weight of the hurt you are carrying, little irritants seem like massive sins. You try to avoid making eye contact and stay occupied and busy yourself. The nights are lonely as you turn away from one another and sleep apart.

You mentally compile a list of your spouse's mistakes and betrayals. The disputes that erupt suddenly include the same tired accusations and justifications. You're yearning in your heart for a sincere apology. I apologize for breaking the ice between us.

You and your partner could feel as if a high wall is standing between you right now. Nobody wants to dismantle the foundation on which the first brick was laid. However, you really have a

large sledgehammer in your hand. Reconnect
with one another with the force of confession.

Truth is invited to your wedding by confession.
It makes the decision quite honest, stating, "This
was the terrible choice I made. This was my
egotistical goal. My actions, words, and attitudes
affected you and our relationship. These are the
ways that I didn't properly adore you. I know it
was bad because of how I hurt others in this way.
As you own your mistake and accept
responsibility for the result, confession bares
you. No lying, no minimizing, and no
justifications.

The door to reconciliation is opened by
confession.
It moves bravely closer to the person you adore.
Rebuilding trust via confession and humbly
pleading for compassion "I ache because I
wounded you," it declares. It enables your hurt
loved one to experience hearing and
understanding. As you both make the decision to
go ahead in a better manner, teamwork emerges.

Your partner discovers a secure environment to discuss whatever sort of consolation and assurance is required. There is a glimmer of hope that your love may be reignited.

Confessional Can Help You Heal.
When handled graciously, the relationship is repaired. Because you are sure of receiving forgiveness and cleansing when you confess your sins to God. (1 John 1:9) It leaves the past in the past and frees you from regret, shame, and secrets. Your souls will benefit from the delicious medicine of my sincere apologies, which will help you move closer to the lovely unity that God intended for you to know.

Today, incline your hearts to one another and express your regret. Offer one another forgiveness and a genuine, real confession. Discover relief from regret, humiliation, and guilt. Take kindness in each other's arms. Allow God to perform a miraculous healing to restore intimacy and joy to your marriage.

So that you might get healing, confess your
faults to one another and pray for one another.
(James 5:16)

CHAPTER SIX

ALWAYS TOUCH

Touch may be a potent non-verbal tool for expressing feelings. It provides a subtler and more complex way of interacting with people. Touch, whether it be a hug or a pat on the back, may express uplifting feelings of love and thanks. Making eye contact is another crucial component of expressing compassion. An arm over someone's shoulder, for instance, may sometimes be more consoling than words when they are grieving.

Negative emotions may also be conveyed via touch or hesitancy in contact. Imagine a parent firmly squeezing their child's hand as they are both holding hands. This circumstance could notify the youngster that their caregiver is afraid and alert them to it. A protracted embrace is an example of a more personal kind of contact that requires safety and connection. People often pick up on whether someone is uneasy or unresponsive to that type of contact. When used in conjunction with speech, eye contact, and body language, touch has the ability to deepen communication.

With your partner, practice the idea of meaningful contact!

A marriage has to have the same kind of deep physical contact that we witness in our children.

One smart husband recognized the significance of this need during a trying period his wife was going through, and it was the best thing he could have done to minister to her.

One morning, while Marilyn was getting ready, she became aware of something that didn't feel quite right. She did not know she had a little bump on her breast until she felt it.

Although Marilyn didn't have a lot of concerns, she was aware enough from reading publications and watching television to realize that she should get it examined. She contacted the doctor to schedule an appointment after telling her husband, Art, what she planned to do. Marilyn saw the doctor two weeks later to have the lump biopsied. She was in the hospital bed three days after her visit, where she would soon have a radical mastectomy.

What Art would think of her now was the toughest thing for Marilyn to deal with following the operation, not her recuperation. Would he still find her attractive? What would he think if he touched her? These and other inquiries kept repeating in her head.

Marilyn and Art were the only people in her room on the day she was scheduled for discharge from the hospital. Her spouse grabbed her hands in his and sat down on her bed.

I want you to know something, Sugar, he said. I still think you're gorgeous, just like the night of our wedding. Never forget that, please.

When the door was shut, Art gave her a wink and added, "After you go home and have a chance to recover, we're going to have to have the lock changed on the door."

While giving her husband a hug, Marilyn started crying. She understood precisely what he meant by his last remark. One of their lads had entered their room at a very inopportune moment early on in their marriage because someone had failed to shut the door. The following day, a new lock was put on the door as a consequence. Their secret code for a quiet evening was "We're going to have to have the lock repaired on the door."

Marilyn had been worried about how Art would treat her outside of the bedroom as well as how the procedure would influence their sexual connection. She was reassured by his words and deeds that morning that this crucial aspect of the blessing would continue to exist in their relationship.

In a developing relationship, physical contact is essential, but it shouldn't be the only time a couple touches. In his book, Sex Begins in the Kitchen, real closeness grows out of little things like touching in the kitchen, strolling hand in hand through a mall, or cuddling up next to each other on the couch while watching TV.

Speaking of "sex starting in the kitchen," a recent seminar attendee told us a genuine tale about how he attempted to use the idea of meaningful contact with his wife and ended up in an awkward scenario.

The idea of meaningful contact really remained with this individual after hearing it discussed repeatedly. He came inside one day to freshen up and take a shower after mowing the lawn. After finishing his shower, he went over to the towel rack to get a towel since he had left the bedroom door open. He could see his wife standing in the kitchen, putting the finishing touches on their supper.

What a moment for heartfelt touching, he reflected. He hurried down the hallway in his birthday suit and rushed into the kitchen to give his wife a hearty embrace without giving it a second's notice. His neighbor's wife had been over to chat, but he was unable to see her from the bedroom or as he hurried down the hallway. When it came to this husband, that surprised neighbor got a much bigger surprise than she could have imagined!No one could blame him for his commitment to meaningfully touching his wife, even if his timing was horrible!

Your relationships may benefit greatly from meaningful contact in many ways. According to Psychology Today, regardless of gender, individuals who were comfortable with touching tended to be more emotionally unstable and socially distant. In contrast, those who were uncomfortable with contact tended to be chatty, upbeat, socially dominant, and nonconforming.

People who were more at ease with touch were less wary of other people's intents and motivations and had less anxiety and stress in their daily lives.

Despite its strength, touch cannot support a blossoming marriage on its own. Three intimacy measures were employed by researchers at the University of Illinois to assess marital pleasure and satisfaction. They discovered that each kind of closeness had a valuable contribution of its own. However, the absence of the last two components of the blessing—emotional and verbal intimacy—was most strongly associated with the likelihood of conflict and divorce. It's crucial to keep in constant contact if you want to develop greater closeness in your marriage.

CHAPTER SEVEN
PRAY TOGETHER

Marriages are strengthened via joint prayer, which is also a means of seeking God's guidance. That discipline then strengthens and grows the marriage as you pray and reach agreements on issues. Additionally, you may battle for your marriage through prayer when tough times arise.

Since marriage is more spiritual than physical, intimacy cannot be fully realized if it merely occurs naturally. You must also maintain the fire together on the altar of prayer. Prayer is essential because it is essential for the fulfillment of the goal for which God created two people to become one, which goes beyond the enjoyment and contentment of the couple. Be thoughtful about it.

Together, create a prayer plan and work on it.

What do we do as a couple when we pray together now that we have a strategy in place? The significance of praying for one another is a fundamental principle to bear in mind. While the Bible does not specifically state that husbands and wives should pray for one another, James 5:16 does state that we should "pray for each other so that you may be cured." That undoubtedly includes wives praying for husbands and husbands praying for spouses. One married couple remarked that every time we pray together, we start by saying a blessing over each other. We do this to uplift and reassure our partner. One of the things we do is agree to pray for each other by finding various prayers in the Bible. One of our favorites is a prayer Paul said for the Philippians in Philippians 1:9-10.In his letter, he prayed that his love would grow in wisdom and depth of understanding, enabling him to see the appropriate course of action and remain pure and spotless until the coming of Christ.

Pray in silence as a group. Too often, couples mistakenly think that they can only pray together aloud. It's important to keep in mind that group prayer is the key. When discussing this with couples' groups, we advise them to start by saying a quiet prayer. The rules are as follows: First, take a seat side by side and hold hands. Many couples have mentioned how crucial it was to be touching one another as they prayed. Next, discuss some of your shared worries as a pair. One of you should say to the other, "Let's pray about these topics," as you wrap up the chat. Finally, take some time to pray silently as a group. Whoever completes the task first should grip their partner's hand to signal, "I've done it." The other individual squeezes back once they're done. Congratulations! You just prayed as a group. After repeating this repeatedly, you could eventually end by saying "Amen" aloud, squeezing your partner's hand, and waiting for them to respond.

Recite the last quiet prayer. The second way you could pray with one another is an extension of the first.It advances our progress toward more openness and comfort in our joint prayer. Instead of just saying, "Amen," to close your quiet prayer, decide that the other person will finish their silent prayer out loud after a hand squeeze. This need not be a deep statement. Simply express your gratitude and appreciation for the understanding that God is with you, that he not only hears your prayers but also understands and hears the deeper needs of your soul, or thank God for being with you in both your conversation and prayer times.

Write down your supplication. First, compose a brief, straightforward prayer that has significance for you. Keep your partner out of this. Once everyone is present, read your spouse your prayer. After you've both done, you may want to chat about how God has answered each other's prayers and how it feels to hear each other speak to Him. You may also read aloud a few of the prayers that are supplied at the conclusion of each chapter.

Pray as you speak. By taking a step back and intentionally bringing God into the dialogue, we may pray together in this way. You might just pause your talking as a couple and offer, "Let's pray about this for a bit." If you are still in the group prayer stage and are not speaking, pray in silence about what you have just discussed.Simply accept that God is there in your dialogue while you are speaking your prayers aloud. For instance, one of us may only say, "Lord, you are here listening as we chat, and we want to recognize your presence and pray for your assistance with this circumstance," while we are discussing a worry we have. Even this may be made more concise, or the other person can add a few more sentences to their prayer. When we do this, we seldom utter the word "Amen"; instead, we just resume talking. You'll gradually start to talk about God more naturally and become more conscious of his presence.

Every day, they pray aloud together.The only difference between this and our prior advice is that you are now sufficiently used to the procedure that you may express your prayer aloud in front of your partner. In our survey, we asked couples how they transitioned from praying aloud to praying quietly together (i.e., was it challenging?). We were curious as to whether or not couples discussed it in advance or whether it simply occurred. We were taken aback when some of them—including the pair we previously mentioned—replied, "We opened our lips and said..." We chuckled, but it really does come down to that strategy—speaking out what we are asking for from God in our hearts. Our nighttime prayer session has been extended to other times of the day as we have become more used to speaking our prayers aloud together over the years. One of us may feel the need to pray while we are together, so we pause and do so. Despite the fact that we still consciously pause to pray as a group, it is now more of a natural aspect of our discourse.

Prayer should be "vulnerable." When we speak about praying together, we believe the majority of men (and some spouses) are afraid of this kind of prayer. It is challenging, and we definitely don't advise beginning in this manner. When we pray in a vulnerable way, we do it in front of our partner. We also pray, "Lord, help me," in addition to "Lord, assist us" and "Lord, help them." When we pray in this fashion, we feel comfortable enough with one another to bring our flaws, mistakes, and challenges in front of the other person while being honest and open with God. The reason this kind of group prayer is mentioned last is not because it is the greatest, but rather because it is the most challenging. Some couples may never pray together in this manner, while others may get used to doing so and believe that doing so significantly increases their spiritual connection. But keep in mind, the objective isn't to pray vulnerably with one another; it's only to pray regularly with one another.